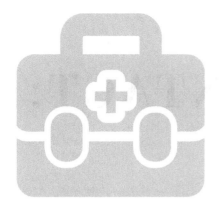

MEDICATION LOGBOOK

MW00872537

This book belongs to:

👤 _____

📍 _____

📞 _____

Emergency Contact

_____

_____

DOCTOR'S CONTACT:

Name		Hospital	
Email		Phone	
Address			
Notes			

Name		Hospital	
Email		Phone	
Address			
Notes			

Name		Hospital	
Email		Phone	
Address			
Notes			

Name		Hospital	
Email		Phone	
Address			
Notes			

Name		Hospital	
Email		Phone	
Address			
Notes			

Week Start: _____

Week finish: _____

Medication	Dosage	Time	Mon	Tues	Wed	Thurs	Fri	Sat	Sun
		A.M Noon P.M Bedtime							

Medication	Dosage	Time	Mon	Tues	Wed	Thurs	Fri	Sat	Sun
		A.M Noon P.M Bedtime							

Medication	Dosage	Time	Mon	Tues	Wed	Thurs	Fri	Sat	Sun
		A.M Noon P.M Bedtime							

Medication	Dosage	Time	Mon	Tues	Wed	Thurs	Fri	Sat	Sun
		A.M Noon P.M Bedtime							

Medication	Dosage	Time	Mon	Tues	Wed	Thurs	Fri	Sat	Sun
		A.M Noon P.M Bedtime							

Medication	Dosage	Time	Mon	Tues	Wed	Thurs	Fri	Sat	Sun
		A.M Noon P.M Bedtime							

NOTES & DAILY DETAILS

Week Start: _____

Week finish: _____

Medication	Dosage	Time	Mon	Tues	Wed	Thurs	Fri	Sat	Sun
		A.M							
		Noon							
		P.M							
		Bedtime							

Medication	Dosage	Time	Mon	Tues	Wed	Thurs	Fri	Sat	Sun
		A.M							
		Noon							
		P.M							
		Bedtime							

Medication	Dosage	Time	Mon	Tues	Wed	Thurs	Fri	Sat	Sun
		A.M							
		Noon							
		P.M							
		Bedtime							

Medication	Dosage	Time	Mon	Tues	Wed	Thurs	Fri	Sat	Sun
		A.M							
		Noon							
		P.M							
		Bedtime							

Medication	Dosage	Time	Mon	Tues	Wed	Thurs	Fri	Sat	Sun
		A.M							
		Noon							
		P.M							
		Bedtime							

Medication	Dosage	Time	Mon	Tues	Wed	Thurs	Fri	Sat	Sun
		A.M							
		Noon							
		P.M							
		Bedtime							

Medication	Dosage	Time	Mon	Tues	Wed	Thurs	Fri	Sat	Sun
		A.M Noon P.M Bedtime							

Medication	Dosage	Time	Mon	Tues	Wed	Thurs	Fri	Sat	Sun
		A.M Noon P.M Bedtime							

Medication	Dosage	Time	Mon	Tues	Wed	Thurs	Fri	Sat	Sun
		A.M Noon P.M Bedtime							

Medication	Dosage	Time	Mon	Tues	Wed	Thurs	Fri	Sat	Sun
		A.M Noon P.M Bedtime							

Medication	Dosage	Time	Mon	Tues	Wed	Thurs	Fri	Sat	Sun
		A.M Noon P.M Bedtime							

Medication	Dosage	Time	Mon	Tues	Wed	Thurs	Fri	Sat	Sun
		A.M Noon P.M Bedtime							

NOTES & DAILY DETAILS

Week Start:_____

Week finish:_____

Medication	Dosage	Time	Mon	Tues	Wed	Thurs	Fri	Sat	Sun
		A.M							
		Noon							
		P.M							
		Bedtime							

Medication	Dosage	Time	Mon	Tues	Wed	Thurs	Fri	Sat	Sun
		A.M							
		Noon							
		P.M							
		Bedtime							

Medication	Dosage	Time	Mon	Tues	Wed	Thurs	Fri	Sat	Sun
		A.M							
		Noon							
		P.M							
		Bedtime							

Medication	Dosage	Time	Mon	Tues	Wed	Thurs	Fri	Sat	Sun
		A.M							
		Noon							
		P.M							
		Bedtime							

Medication	Dosage	Time	Mon	Tues	Wed	Thurs	Fri	Sat	Sun
		A.M							
		Noon							
		P.M							
		Bedtime							

Medication	Dosage	Time	Mon	Tues	Wed	Thurs	Fri	Sat	Sun
		A.M							
		Noon							
		P.M							
		Bedtime							

Week Start: _____

Week finish: _____

Medication	Dosage	Time	Mon	Tues	Wed	Thurs	Fri	Sat	Sun
		A.M							
		Noon							
		P.M							
		Bedtime							

Medication	Dosage	Time	Mon	Tues	Wed	Thurs	Fri	Sat	Sun
		A.M							
		Noon							
		P.M							
		Bedtime							

Medication	Dosage	Time	Mon	Tues	Wed	Thurs	Fri	Sat	Sun
		A.M							
		Noon							
		P.M							
		Bedtime							

Medication	Dosage	Time	Mon	Tues	Wed	Thurs	Fri	Sat	Sun
		A.M							
		Noon							
		P.M							
		Bedtime							

Medication	Dosage	Time	Mon	Tues	Wed	Thurs	Fri	Sat	Sun
		A.M							
		Noon							
		P.M							
		Bedtime							

Medication	Dosage	Time	Mon	Tues	Wed	Thurs	Fri	Sat	Sun
		A.M							
		Noon							
		P.M							
		Bedtime							

Week Start: _____

Week finish: _____

Medication	Dosage	Time	Mon	Tues	Wed	Thurs	Fri	Sat	Sun
		A.M Noon P.M Bedtime							

Medication	Dosage	Time	Mon	Tues	Wed	Thurs	Fri	Sat	Sun
		A.M Noon P.M Bedtime							

Medication	Dosage	Time	Mon	Tues	Wed	Thurs	Fri	Sat	Sun
		A.M Noon P.M Bedtime							

Medication	Dosage	Time	Mon	Tues	Wed	Thurs	Fri	Sat	Sun
		A.M Noon P.M Bedtime							

Medication	Dosage	Time	Mon	Tues	Wed	Thurs	Fri	Sat	Sun
		A.M Noon P.M Bedtime							

Medication	Dosage	Time	Mon	Tues	Wed	Thurs	Fri	Sat	Sun
		A.M Noon P.M Bedtime							

NOTES & DAILY DETAILS

Medication	Dosage	Time	Mon	Tues	Wed	Thurs	Fri	Sat	Sun
		A.M							
		Noon							
		P.M							
		Bedtime							

Medication	Dosage	Time	Mon	Tues	Wed	Thurs	Fri	Sat	Sun
		A.M							
		Noon							
		P.M							
		Bedtime							

Medication	Dosage	Time	Mon	Tues	Wed	Thurs	Fri	Sat	Sun
		A.M							
		Noon							
		P.M							
		Bedtime							

Medication	Dosage	Time	Mon	Tues	Wed	Thurs	Fri	Sat	Sun
		A.M							
		Noon							
		P.M							
		Bedtime							

Medication	Dosage	Time	Mon	Tues	Wed	Thurs	Fri	Sat	Sun
		A.M							
		Noon							
		P.M							
		Bedtime							

Medication	Dosage	Time	Mon	Tues	Wed	Thurs	Fri	Sat	Sun
		A.M							
		Noon							
		P.M							
		Bedtime							

NOTES & DAILY DETAILS

Medication	Dosage	Time	Mon	Tues	Wed	Thurs	Fri	Sat	Sun
		A.M							
		Noon							
		P.M							
		Bedtime							

Medication	Dosage	Time	Mon	Tues	Wed	Thurs	Fri	Sat	Sun
		A.M							
		Noon							
		P.M							
		Bedtime							

Medication	Dosage	Time	Mon	Tues	Wed	Thurs	Fri	Sat	Sun
		A.M							
		Noon							
		P.M							
		Bedtime							

Medication	Dosage	Time	Mon	Tues	Wed	Thurs	Fri	Sat	Sun
		A.M							
		Noon							
		P.M							
		Bedtime							

Medication	Dosage	Time	Mon	Tues	Wed	Thurs	Fri	Sat	Sun
		A.M							
		Noon							
		P.M							
		Bedtime							

Medication	Dosage	Time	Mon	Tues	Wed	Thurs	Fri	Sat	Sun
		A.M							
		Noon							
		P.M							
		Bedtime							

Medication	Dosage	Time	Mon	Tues	Wed	Thurs	Fri	Sat	Sun
		A.M Noon P.M Bedtime							

Medication	Dosage	Time	Mon	Tues	Wed	Thurs	Fri	Sat	Sun
		A.M Noon P.M Bedtime							

Medication	Dosage	Time	Mon	Tues	Wed	Thurs	Fri	Sat	Sun
		A.M Noon P.M Bedtime							

Medication	Dosage	Time	Mon	Tues	Wed	Thurs	Fri	Sat	Sun
		A.M Noon P.M Bedtime							

Medication	Dosage	Time	Mon	Tues	Wed	Thurs	Fri	Sat	Sun
		A.M Noon P.M Bedtime							

Medication	Dosage	Time	Mon	Tues	Wed	Thurs	Fri	Sat	Sun
		A.M Noon P.M Bedtime							

NOTES & DAILY DETAILS

Medication	Dosage	Time	Mon	Tues	Wed	Thurs	Fri	Sat	Sun
		A.M							
		Noon							
		P.M							
		Bedtime							

Medication	Dosage	Time	Mon	Tues	Wed	Thurs	Fri	Sat	Sun
		A.M							
		Noon							
		P.M							
		Bedtime							

Medication	Dosage	Time	Mon	Tues	Wed	Thurs	Fri	Sat	Sun
		A.M							
		Noon							
		P.M							
		Bedtime							

Medication	Dosage	Time	Mon	Tues	Wed	Thurs	Fri	Sat	Sun
		A.M							
		Noon							
		P.M							
		Bedtime							

Medication	Dosage	Time	Mon	Tues	Wed	Thurs	Fri	Sat	Sun
		A.M							
		Noon							
		P.M							
		Bedtime							

Medication	Dosage	Time	Mon	Tues	Wed	Thurs	Fri	Sat	Sun
		A.M							
		Noon							
		P.M							
		Bedtime							

NOTES & DAILY DETAILS

Week Start: _____

Week finish: _____

Medication	Dosage	Time	Mon	Tues	Wed	Thurs	Fri	Sat	Sun
		A.M							
		Noon							
		P.M							
		Bedtime							

Medication	Dosage	Time	Mon	Tues	Wed	Thurs	Fri	Sat	Sun
		A.M							
		Noon							
		P.M							
		Bedtime							

Medication	Dosage	Time	Mon	Tues	Wed	Thurs	Fri	Sat	Sun
		A.M							
		Noon							
		P.M							
		Bedtime							

Medication	Dosage	Time	Mon	Tues	Wed	Thurs	Fri	Sat	Sun
		A.M							
		Noon							
		P.M							
		Bedtime							

Medication	Dosage	Time	Mon	Tues	Wed	Thurs	Fri	Sat	Sun
		A.M							
		Noon							
		P.M							
		Bedtime							

Medication	Dosage	Time	Mon	Tues	Wed	Thurs	Fri	Sat	Sun
		A.M							
		Noon							
		P.M							
		Bedtime							

NOTES & DAILY DETAILS

Week Start: _____

Week finish: _____

Medication	Dosage	Time	Mon	Tues	Wed	Thurs	Fri	Sat	Sun
		A.M Noon P.M Bedtime							

Medication	Dosage	Time	Mon	Tues	Wed	Thurs	Fri	Sat	Sun
		A.M Noon P.M Bedtime							

Medication	Dosage	Time	Mon	Tues	Wed	Thurs	Fri	Sat	Sun
		A.M Noon P.M Bedtime							

Medication	Dosage	Time	Mon	Tues	Wed	Thurs	Fri	Sat	Sun
		A.M Noon P.M Bedtime							

Medication	Dosage	Time	Mon	Tues	Wed	Thurs	Fri	Sat	Sun
		A.M Noon P.M Bedtime							

Medication	Dosage	Time	Mon	Tues	Wed	Thurs	Fri	Sat	Sun
		A.M Noon P.M Bedtime							

NOTES & DAILY DETAILS

Week Start: _____

Week finish: _____

Medication	Dosage	Time	Mon	Tues	Wed	Thurs	Fri	Sat	Sun
		A.M							
		Noon							
		P.M							
		Bedtime							

Medication	Dosage	Time	Mon	Tues	Wed	Thurs	Fri	Sat	Sun
		A.M							
		Noon							
		P.M							
		Bedtime							

Medication	Dosage	Time	Mon	Tues	Wed	Thurs	Fri	Sat	Sun
		A.M							
		Noon							
		P.M							
		Bedtime							

Medication	Dosage	Time	Mon	Tues	Wed	Thurs	Fri	Sat	Sun
		A.M							
		Noon							
		P.M							
		Bedtime							

Medication	Dosage	Time	Mon	Tues	Wed	Thurs	Fri	Sat	Sun
		A.M							
		Noon							
		P.M							
		Bedtime							

Medication	Dosage	Time	Mon	Tues	Wed	Thurs	Fri	Sat	Sun
		A.M							
		Noon							
		P.M							
		Bedtime							

NOTES & DAILY DETAILS

Medication	Dosage	Time	Mon	Tues	Wed	Thurs	Fri	Sat	Sun
		A.M Noon P.M Bedtime							

Medication	Dosage	Time	Mon	Tues	Wed	Thurs	Fri	Sat	Sun
		A.M Noon P.M Bedtime							

Medication	Dosage	Time	Mon	Tues	Wed	Thurs	Fri	Sat	Sun
		A.M Noon P.M Bedtime							

Medication	Dosage	Time	Mon	Tues	Wed	Thurs	Fri	Sat	Sun
		A.M Noon P.M Bedtime							

Medication	Dosage	Time	Mon	Tues	Wed	Thurs	Fri	Sat	Sun
		A.M Noon P.M Bedtime							

Medication	Dosage	Time	Mon	Tues	Wed	Thurs	Fri	Sat	Sun
		A.M Noon P.M Bedtime							

NOTES & DAILY DETAILS

Week Start: _____

Week finish: _____

Medication	Dosage	Time	Mon	Tues	Wed	Thurs	Fri	Sat	Sun
		A.M							
		Noon							
		P.M							
		Bedtime							

Medication	Dosage	Time	Mon	Tues	Wed	Thurs	Fri	Sat	Sun
		A.M							
		Noon							
		P.M							
		Bedtime							

Medication	Dosage	Time	Mon	Tues	Wed	Thurs	Fri	Sat	Sun
		A.M							
		Noon							
		P.M							
		Bedtime							

Medication	Dosage	Time	Mon	Tues	Wed	Thurs	Fri	Sat	Sun
		A.M							
		Noon							
		P.M							
		Bedtime							

Medication	Dosage	Time	Mon	Tues	Wed	Thurs	Fri	Sat	Sun
		A.M							
		Noon							
		P.M							
		Bedtime							

Medication	Dosage	Time	Mon	Tues	Wed	Thurs	Fri	Sat	Sun
		A.M							
		Noon							
		P.M							
		Bedtime							

Week Start: _____

Week finish: _____

Medication	Dosage	Time	Mon	Tues	Wed	Thurs	Fri	Sat	Sun
		A.M							
		Noon							
		P.M							
		Bedtime							

Medication	Dosage	Time	Mon	Tues	Wed	Thurs	Fri	Sat	Sun
		A.M							
		Noon							
		P.M							
		Bedtime							

Medication	Dosage	Time	Mon	Tues	Wed	Thurs	Fri	Sat	Sun
		A.M							
		Noon							
		P.M							
		Bedtime							

Medication	Dosage	Time	Mon	Tues	Wed	Thurs	Fri	Sat	Sun
		A.M							
		Noon							
		P.M							
		Bedtime							

Medication	Dosage	Time	Mon	Tues	Wed	Thurs	Fri	Sat	Sun
		A.M							
		Noon							
		P.M							
		Bedtime							

Medication	Dosage	Time	Mon	Tues	Wed	Thurs	Fri	Sat	Sun
		A.M							
		Noon							
		P.M							
		Bedtime							

NOTES & DAILY DETAILS

Medication	Dosage	Time	Mon	Tues	Wed	Thurs	Fri	Sat	Sun
		A.M Noon P.M Bedtime							

Medication	Dosage	Time	Mon	Tues	Wed	Thurs	Fri	Sat	Sun
		A.M Noon P.M Bedtime							

Medication	Dosage	Time	Mon	Tues	Wed	Thurs	Fri	Sat	Sun
		A.M Noon P.M Bedtime							

Medication	Dosage	Time	Mon	Tues	Wed	Thurs	Fri	Sat	Sun
		A.M Noon P.M Bedtime							

Medication	Dosage	Time	Mon	Tues	Wed	Thurs	Fri	Sat	Sun
		A.M Noon P.M Bedtime							

Medication	Dosage	Time	Mon	Tues	Wed	Thurs	Fri	Sat	Sun
		A.M Noon P.M Bedtime							

Week Start:
Week finish:

Medication	Dosage	Time	Mon	Tues	Wed	Thurs	Fri	Sat	Sun
		A.M							
		Noon							
		P.M							
		Bedtime							

Medication	Dosage	Time	Mon	Tues	Wed	Thurs	Fri	Sat	Sun
		A.M							
		Noon							
		P.M							
		Bedtime							

Medication	Dosage	Time	Mon	Tues	Wed	Thurs	Fri	Sat	Sun
		A.M							
		Noon							
		P.M							
		Bedtime							

Medication	Dosage	Time	Mon	Tues	Wed	Thurs	Fri	Sat	Sun
		A.M							
		Noon							
		P.M							
		Bedtime							

Medication	Dosage	Time	Mon	Tues	Wed	Thurs	Fri	Sat	Sun
		A.M							
		Noon							
		P.M							
		Bedtime							

Medication	Dosage	Time	Mon	Tues	Wed	Thurs	Fri	Sat	Sun
		A.M							
		Noon							
		P.M							
		Bedtime							

Week Start: _____

Week finish: _____

Medication	Dosage	Time	Mon	Tues	Wed	Thurs	Fri	Sat	Sun
		A.M Noon P.M Bedtime							

Medication	Dosage	Time	Mon	Tues	Wed	Thurs	Fri	Sat	Sun
		A.M Noon P.M Bedtime							

Medication	Dosage	Time	Mon	Tues	Wed	Thurs	Fri	Sat	Sun
		A.M Noon P.M Bedtime							

Medication	Dosage	Time	Mon	Tues	Wed	Thurs	Fri	Sat	Sun
		A.M Noon P.M Bedtime							

Medication	Dosage	Time	Mon	Tues	Wed	Thurs	Fri	Sat	Sun
		A.M Noon P.M Bedtime							

Medication	Dosage	Time	Mon	Tues	Wed	Thurs	Fri	Sat	Sun
		A.M Noon P.M Bedtime							

Week Start: _____

Week finish: _____

Medication	Dosage	Time	Mon	Tues	Wed	Thurs	Fri	Sat	Sun
		A.M Noon P.M Bedtime							

Medication	Dosage	Time	Mon	Tues	Wed	Thurs	Fri	Sat	Sun
		A.M Noon P.M Bedtime							

Medication	Dosage	Time	Mon	Tues	Wed	Thurs	Fri	Sat	Sun
		A.M Noon P.M Bedtime							

Medication	Dosage	Time	Mon	Tues	Wed	Thurs	Fri	Sat	Sun
		A.M Noon P.M Bedtime							

Medication	Dosage	Time	Mon	Tues	Wed	Thurs	Fri	Sat	Sun
		A.M Noon P.M Bedtime							

Medication	Dosage	Time	Mon	Tues	Wed	Thurs	Fri	Sat	Sun
		A.M Noon P.M Bedtime							

Week Start: _____

Week finish: _____

Medication	Dosage	Time	Mon	Tues	Wed	Thurs	Fri	Sat	Sun
		A.M							
		Noon							
		P.M							
		Bedtime							

Medication	Dosage	Time	Mon	Tues	Wed	Thurs	Fri	Sat	Sun
		A.M							
		Noon							
		P.M							
		Bedtime							

Medication	Dosage	Time	Mon	Tues	Wed	Thurs	Fri	Sat	Sun
		A.M							
		Noon							
		P.M							
		Bedtime							

Medication	Dosage	Time	Mon	Tues	Wed	Thurs	Fri	Sat	Sun
		A.M							
		Noon							
		P.M							
		Bedtime							

Medication	Dosage	Time	Mon	Tues	Wed	Thurs	Fri	Sat	Sun
		A.M							
		Noon							
		P.M							
		Bedtime							

Medication	Dosage	Time	Mon	Tues	Wed	Thurs	Fri	Sat	Sun
		A.M							
		Noon							
		P.M							
		Bedtime							

Medication	Dosage	Time	Mon	Tues	Wed	Thurs	Fri	Sat	Sun
		A.M							
		Noon							
		P.M							
		Bedtime							

Medication	Dosage	Time	Mon	Tues	Wed	Thurs	Fri	Sat	Sun
		A.M							
		Noon							
		P.M							
		Bedtime							

Medication	Dosage	Time	Mon	Tues	Wed	Thurs	Fri	Sat	Sun
		A.M							
		Noon							
		P.M							
		Bedtime							

Medication	Dosage	Time	Mon	Tues	Wed	Thurs	Fri	Sat	Sun
		A.M							
		Noon							
		P.M							
		Bedtime							

Medication	Dosage	Time	Mon	Tues	Wed	Thurs	Fri	Sat	Sun
		A.M							
		Noon							
		P.M							
		Bedtime							

Medication	Dosage	Time	Mon	Tues	Wed	Thurs	Fri	Sat	Sun
		A.M							
		Noon							
		P.M							
		Bedtime							

NOTES & DAILY DETAILS

Week Start: _____

Week finish: _____

Medication	Dosage	Time	Mon	Tues	Wed	Thurs	Fri	Sat	Sun
		A.M							
		Noon							
		P.M							
		Bedtime							

Medication	Dosage	Time	Mon	Tues	Wed	Thurs	Fri	Sat	Sun
		A.M							
		Noon							
		P.M							
		Bedtime							

Medication	Dosage	Time	Mon	Tues	Wed	Thurs	Fri	Sat	Sun
		A.M							
		Noon							
		P.M							
		Bedtime							

Medication	Dosage	Time	Mon	Tues	Wed	Thurs	Fri	Sat	Sun
		A.M							
		Noon							
		P.M							
		Bedtime							

Medication	Dosage	Time	Mon	Tues	Wed	Thurs	Fri	Sat	Sun
		A.M							
		Noon							
		P.M							
		Bedtime							

Medication	Dosage	Time	Mon	Tues	Wed	Thurs	Fri	Sat	Sun
		A.M							
		Noon							
		P.M							
		Bedtime							

NOTES & DAILY DETAILS

<table>
<tr><td></td><td></td><td></td></tr>
</table>

Week Start: _____

Week finish: _____

Medication	Dosage	Time	Mon	Tues	Wed	Thurs	Fri	Sat	Sun
		A.M Noon P.M Bedtime							

Medication	Dosage	Time	Mon	Tues	Wed	Thurs	Fri	Sat	Sun
		A.M Noon P.M Bedtime							

Medication	Dosage	Time	Mon	Tues	Wed	Thurs	Fri	Sat	Sun
		A.M Noon P.M Bedtime							

Medication	Dosage	Time	Mon	Tues	Wed	Thurs	Fri	Sat	Sun
		A.M Noon P.M Bedtime							

Medication	Dosage	Time	Mon	Tues	Wed	Thurs	Fri	Sat	Sun
		A.M Noon P.M Bedtime							

Medication	Dosage	Time	Mon	Tues	Wed	Thurs	Fri	Sat	Sun
		A.M Noon P.M Bedtime							

NOTES & DAILY DETAILS

Week Start: _____

Week finish: _____

Medication	Dosage	Time	Mon	Tues	Wed	Thurs	Fri	Sat	Sun
		A.M							
		Noon							
		P.M							
		Bedtime							

Medication	Dosage	Time	Mon	Tues	Wed	Thurs	Fri	Sat	Sun
		A.M							
		Noon							
		P.M							
		Bedtime							

Medication	Dosage	Time	Mon	Tues	Wed	Thurs	Fri	Sat	Sun
		A.M							
		Noon							
		P.M							
		Bedtime							

Medication	Dosage	Time	Mon	Tues	Wed	Thurs	Fri	Sat	Sun
		A.M							
		Noon							
		P.M							
		Bedtime							

Medication	Dosage	Time	Mon	Tues	Wed	Thurs	Fri	Sat	Sun
		A.M							
		Noon							
		P.M							
		Bedtime							

Medication	Dosage	Time	Mon	Tues	Wed	Thurs	Fri	Sat	Sun
		A.M							
		Noon							
		P.M							
		Bedtime							

Medication	Dosage	Time	Mon	Tues	Wed	Thurs	Fri	Sat	Sun
		A.M							
		Noon							
		P.M							
		Bedtime							

Medication	Dosage	Time	Mon	Tues	Wed	Thurs	Fri	Sat	Sun
		A.M							
		Noon							
		P.M							
		Bedtime							

Medication	Dosage	Time	Mon	Tues	Wed	Thurs	Fri	Sat	Sun
		A.M							
		Noon							
		P.M							
		Bedtime							

Medication	Dosage	Time	Mon	Tues	Wed	Thurs	Fri	Sat	Sun
		A.M							
		Noon							
		P.M							
		Bedtime							

Medication	Dosage	Time	Mon	Tues	Wed	Thurs	Fri	Sat	Sun
		A.M							
		Noon							
		P.M							
		Bedtime							

Medication	Dosage	Time	Mon	Tues	Wed	Thurs	Fri	Sat	Sun
		A.M							
		Noon							
		P.M							
		Bedtime							

Medication	Dosage	Time	Mon	Tues	Wed	Thurs	Fri	Sat	Sun
		A.M Noon P.M Bedtime							

Medication	Dosage	Time	Mon	Tues	Wed	Thurs	Fri	Sat	Sun
		A.M Noon P.M Bedtime							

Medication	Dosage	Time	Mon	Tues	Wed	Thurs	Fri	Sat	Sun
		A.M Noon P.M Bedtime							

Medication	Dosage	Time	Mon	Tues	Wed	Thurs	Fri	Sat	Sun
		A.M Noon P.M Bedtime							

Medication	Dosage	Time	Mon	Tues	Wed	Thurs	Fri	Sat	Sun
		A.M Noon P.M Bedtime							

Medication	Dosage	Time	Mon	Tues	Wed	Thurs	Fri	Sat	Sun
		A.M Noon P.M Bedtime							

NOTES & DAILY DETAILS

Medication	Dosage	Time	Mon	Tues	Wed	Thurs	Fri	Sat	Sun
		A.M							
		Noon							
		P.M							
		Bedtime							

Medication	Dosage	Time	Mon	Tues	Wed	Thurs	Fri	Sat	Sun
		A.M							
		Noon							
		P.M							
		Bedtime							

Medication	Dosage	Time	Mon	Tues	Wed	Thurs	Fri	Sat	Sun
		A.M							
		Noon							
		P.M							
		Bedtime							

Medication	Dosage	Time	Mon	Tues	Wed	Thurs	Fri	Sat	Sun
		A.M							
		Noon							
		P.M							
		Bedtime							

Medication	Dosage	Time	Mon	Tues	Wed	Thurs	Fri	Sat	Sun
		A.M							
		Noon							
		P.M							
		Bedtime							

Medication	Dosage	Time	Mon	Tues	Wed	Thurs	Fri	Sat	Sun
		A.M							
		Noon							
		P.M							
		Bedtime							

NOTES & DAILY DETAILS

Medication	Dosage	Time	Mon	Tues	Wed	Thurs	Fri	Sat	Sun
		A.M Noon P.M Bedtime							

Medication	Dosage	Time	Mon	Tues	Wed	Thurs	Fri	Sat	Sun
		A.M Noon P.M Bedtime							

Medication	Dosage	Time	Mon	Tues	Wed	Thurs	Fri	Sat	Sun
		A.M Noon P.M Bedtime							

Medication	Dosage	Time	Mon	Tues	Wed	Thurs	Fri	Sat	Sun
		A.M Noon P.M Bedtime							

Medication	Dosage	Time	Mon	Tues	Wed	Thurs	Fri	Sat	Sun
		A.M Noon P.M Bedtime							

Medication	Dosage	Time	Mon	Tues	Wed	Thurs	Fri	Sat	Sun
		A.M Noon P.M Bedtime							

NOTES & DAILY DETAILS

Week Start: _____

Week finish: _____

Medication	Dosage	Time	Mon	Tues	Wed	Thurs	Fri	Sat	Sun
		A.M							
		Noon							
		P.M							
		Bedtime							

Medication	Dosage	Time	Mon	Tues	Wed	Thurs	Fri	Sat	Sun
		A.M							
		Noon							
		P.M							
		Bedtime							

Medication	Dosage	Time	Mon	Tues	Wed	Thurs	Fri	Sat	Sun
		A.M							
		Noon							
		P.M							
		Bedtime							

Medication	Dosage	Time	Mon	Tues	Wed	Thurs	Fri	Sat	Sun
		A.M							
		Noon							
		P.M							
		Bedtime							

Medication	Dosage	Time	Mon	Tues	Wed	Thurs	Fri	Sat	Sun
		A.M							
		Noon							
		P.M							
		Bedtime							

Medication	Dosage	Time	Mon	Tues	Wed	Thurs	Fri	Sat	Sun
		A.M							
		Noon							
		P.M							
		Bedtime							

Week Start: _____

Week finish: _____

Medication	Dosage	Time	Mon	Tues	Wed	Thurs	Fri	Sat	Sun
		A.M							
		Noon							
		P.M							
		Bedtime							

Medication	Dosage	Time	Mon	Tues	Wed	Thurs	Fri	Sat	Sun
		A.M							
		Noon							
		P.M							
		Bedtime							

Medication	Dosage	Time	Mon	Tues	Wed	Thurs	Fri	Sat	Sun
		A.M							
		Noon							
		P.M							
		Bedtime							

Medication	Dosage	Time	Mon	Tues	Wed	Thurs	Fri	Sat	Sun
		A.M							
		Noon							
		P.M							
		Bedtime							

Medication	Dosage	Time	Mon	Tues	Wed	Thurs	Fri	Sat	Sun
		A.M							
		Noon							
		P.M							
		Bedtime							

Medication	Dosage	Time	Mon	Tues	Wed	Thurs	Fri	Sat	Sun
		A.M							
		Noon							
		P.M							
		Bedtime							

NOTES & DAILY DETAILS

Week Start: _____

Week finish: _____

Medication	Dosage	Time	Mon	Tues	Wed	Thurs	Fri	Sat	Sun
		A.M Noon P.M Bedtime	☐ ☐ ☐ ☐	☐ ☐ ☐ ☐	☐ ☐ ☐ ☐	☐ ☐ ☐ ☐	☐ ☐ ☐ ☐	☐ ☐ ☐ ☐	☐ ☐ ☐ ☐

Medication	Dosage	Time	Mon	Tues	Wed	Thurs	Fri	Sat	Sun
		A.M Noon P.M Bedtime	☐ ☐ ☐ ☐	☐ ☐ ☐ ☐	☐ ☐ ☐ ☐	☐ ☐ ☐ ☐	☐ ☐ ☐ ☐	☐ ☐ ☐ ☐	☐ ☐ ☐ ☐

Medication	Dosage	Time	Mon	Tues	Wed	Thurs	Fri	Sat	Sun
		A.M Noon P.M Bedtime	☐ ☐ ☐ ☐	☐ ☐ ☐ ☐	☐ ☐ ☐ ☐	☐ ☐ ☐ ☐	☐ ☐ ☐ ☐	☐ ☐ ☐ ☐	☐ ☐ ☐ ☐

Medication	Dosage	Time	Mon	Tues	Wed	Thurs	Fri	Sat	Sun
		A.M Noon P.M Bedtime	☐ ☐ ☐ ☐	☐ ☐ ☐ ☐	☐ ☐ ☐ ☐	☐ ☐ ☐ ☐	☐ ☐ ☐ ☐	☐ ☐ ☐ ☐	☐ ☐ ☐ ☐

Medication	Dosage	Time	Mon	Tues	Wed	Thurs	Fri	Sat	Sun
		A.M Noon P.M Bedtime	☐ ☐ ☐ ☐	☐ ☐ ☐ ☐	☐ ☐ ☐ ☐	☐ ☐ ☐ ☐	☐ ☐ ☐ ☐	☐ ☐ ☐ ☐	☐ ☐ ☐ ☐

Medication	Dosage	Time	Mon	Tues	Wed	Thurs	Fri	Sat	Sun
		A.M Noon P.M Bedtime	☐ ☐ ☐ ☐	☐ ☐ ☐ ☐	☐ ☐ ☐ ☐	☐ ☐ ☐ ☐	☐ ☐ ☐ ☐	☐ ☐ ☐ ☐	☐ ☐ ☐ ☐

NOTES & DAILY DETAILS

Week Start: _____

Week finish: _____

Medication	Dosage	Time	Mon	Tues	Wed	Thurs	Fri	Sat	Sun
		A.M Noon P.M Bedtime							

Medication	Dosage	Time	Mon	Tues	Wed	Thurs	Fri	Sat	Sun
		A.M Noon P.M Bedtime							

Medication	Dosage	Time	Mon	Tues	Wed	Thurs	Fri	Sat	Sun
		A.M Noon P.M Bedtime							

Medication	Dosage	Time	Mon	Tues	Wed	Thurs	Fri	Sat	Sun
		A.M Noon P.M Bedtime							

Medication	Dosage	Time	Mon	Tues	Wed	Thurs	Fri	Sat	Sun
		A.M Noon P.M Bedtime							

Medication	Dosage	Time	Mon	Tues	Wed	Thurs	Fri	Sat	Sun
		A.M Noon P.M Bedtime							

NOTES & DAILY DETAILS

Week Start: _____

Week finish: _____

Medication	Dosage	Time	Mon	Tues	Wed	Thurs	Fri	Sat	Sun
		A.M							
		Noon							
		P.M							
		Bedtime							

Medication	Dosage	Time	Mon	Tues	Wed	Thurs	Fri	Sat	Sun
		A.M							
		Noon							
		P.M							
		Bedtime							

Medication	Dosage	Time	Mon	Tues	Wed	Thurs	Fri	Sat	Sun
		A.M							
		Noon							
		P.M							
		Bedtime							

Medication	Dosage	Time	Mon	Tues	Wed	Thurs	Fri	Sat	Sun
		A.M							
		Noon							
		P.M							
		Bedtime							

Medication	Dosage	Time	Mon	Tues	Wed	Thurs	Fri	Sat	Sun
		A.M							
		Noon							
		P.M							
		Bedtime							

Medication	Dosage	Time	Mon	Tues	Wed	Thurs	Fri	Sat	Sun
		A.M							
		Noon							
		P.M							
		Bedtime							

NOTES & DAILY DETAILS

Medication	Dosage	Time	Mon	Tues	Wed	Thurs	Fri	Sat	Sun
		A.M Noon P.M Bedtime							

Medication	Dosage	Time	Mon	Tues	Wed	Thurs	Fri	Sat	Sun
		A.M Noon P.M Bedtime							

Medication	Dosage	Time	Mon	Tues	Wed	Thurs	Fri	Sat	Sun
		A.M Noon P.M Bedtime							

Medication	Dosage	Time	Mon	Tues	Wed	Thurs	Fri	Sat	Sun
		A.M Noon P.M Bedtime							

Medication	Dosage	Time	Mon	Tues	Wed	Thurs	Fri	Sat	Sun
		A.M Noon P.M Bedtime							

Medication	Dosage	Time	Mon	Tues	Wed	Thurs	Fri	Sat	Sun
		A.M Noon P.M Bedtime							

<table>
<tr><td></td><td></td><td></td><td colspan="7">Week Start: _____

Week finish: _____</td></tr>
</table>

Medication	Dosage	Time	Mon	Tues	Wed	Thurs	Fri	Sat	Sun
		A.M							
		Noon							
		P.M							
		Bedtime							

Medication	Dosage	Time	Mon	Tues	Wed	Thurs	Fri	Sat	Sun
		A.M							
		Noon							
		P.M							
		Bedtime							

Medication	Dosage	Time	Mon	Tues	Wed	Thurs	Fri	Sat	Sun
		A.M							
		Noon							
		P.M							
		Bedtime							

Medication	Dosage	Time	Mon	Tues	Wed	Thurs	Fri	Sat	Sun
		A.M							
		Noon							
		P.M							
		Bedtime							

Medication	Dosage	Time	Mon	Tues	Wed	Thurs	Fri	Sat	Sun
		A.M							
		Noon							
		P.M							
		Bedtime							

Medication	Dosage	Time	Mon	Tues	Wed	Thurs	Fri	Sat	Sun
		A.M							
		Noon							
		P.M							
		Bedtime							

NOTES & DAILY DETAILS

Week Start: _____

Week finish: _____

Medication	Dosage	Time	Mon	Tues	Wed	Thurs	Fri	Sat	Sun
		A.M							
		Noon							
		P.M							
		Bedtime							

Medication	Dosage	Time	Mon	Tues	Wed	Thurs	Fri	Sat	Sun
		A.M							
		Noon							
		P.M							
		Bedtime							

Medication	Dosage	Time	Mon	Tues	Wed	Thurs	Fri	Sat	Sun
		A.M							
		Noon							
		P.M							
		Bedtime							

Medication	Dosage	Time	Mon	Tues	Wed	Thurs	Fri	Sat	Sun
		A.M							
		Noon							
		P.M							
		Bedtime							

Medication	Dosage	Time	Mon	Tues	Wed	Thurs	Fri	Sat	Sun
		A.M							
		Noon							
		P.M							
		Bedtime							

Medication	Dosage	Time	Mon	Tues	Wed	Thurs	Fri	Sat	Sun
		A.M							
		Noon							
		P.M							
		Bedtime							

NOTES & DAILY DETAILS

| Week Start: |
| Week finish: |

Medication	Dosage	Time	Mon	Tues	Wed	Thurs	Fri	Sat	Sun
		A.M							
		Noon							
		P.M							
		Bedtime							

Medication	Dosage	Time	Mon	Tues	Wed	Thurs	Fri	Sat	Sun
		A.M							
		Noon							
		P.M							
		Bedtime							

Medication	Dosage	Time	Mon	Tues	Wed	Thurs	Fri	Sat	Sun
		A.M							
		Noon							
		P.M							
		Bedtime							

Medication	Dosage	Time	Mon	Tues	Wed	Thurs	Fri	Sat	Sun
		A.M							
		Noon							
		P.M							
		Bedtime							

Medication	Dosage	Time	Mon	Tues	Wed	Thurs	Fri	Sat	Sun
		A.M							
		Noon							
		P.M							
		Bedtime							

Medication	Dosage	Time	Mon	Tues	Wed	Thurs	Fri	Sat	Sun
		A.M							
		Noon							
		P.M							
		Bedtime							

NOTES & DAILY DETAILS

| Week Start: _____ |
| Week finish: _____ |

Medication	Dosage	Time	Mon	Tues	Wed	Thurs	Fri	Sat	Sun
		A.M Noon P.M Bedtime							

Medication	Dosage	Time	Mon	Tues	Wed	Thurs	Fri	Sat	Sun
		A.M Noon P.M Bedtime							

Medication	Dosage	Time	Mon	Tues	Wed	Thurs	Fri	Sat	Sun
		A.M Noon P.M Bedtime							

Medication	Dosage	Time	Mon	Tues	Wed	Thurs	Fri	Sat	Sun
		A.M Noon P.M Bedtime							

Medication	Dosage	Time	Mon	Tues	Wed	Thurs	Fri	Sat	Sun
		A.M Noon P.M Bedtime							

Medication	Dosage	Time	Mon	Tues	Wed	Thurs	Fri	Sat	Sun
		A.M Noon P.M Bedtime							

NOTES & DAILY DETAILS

Medication	Dosage	Time	Mon	Tues	Wed	Thurs	Fri	Sat	Sun
		A.M							
		Noon							
		P.M							
		Bedtime							

Medication	Dosage	Time	Mon	Tues	Wed	Thurs	Fri	Sat	Sun
		A.M							
		Noon							
		P.M							
		Bedtime							

Medication	Dosage	Time	Mon	Tues	Wed	Thurs	Fri	Sat	Sun
		A.M							
		Noon							
		P.M							
		Bedtime							

Medication	Dosage	Time	Mon	Tues	Wed	Thurs	Fri	Sat	Sun
		A.M							
		Noon							
		P.M							
		Bedtime							

Medication	Dosage	Time	Mon	Tues	Wed	Thurs	Fri	Sat	Sun
		A.M							
		Noon							
		P.M							
		Bedtime							

Medication	Dosage	Time	Mon	Tues	Wed	Thurs	Fri	Sat	Sun
		A.M							
		Noon							
		P.M							
		Bedtime							

NOTES & DAILY DETAILS

Week Start: _____

Week finish: _____

Medication	Dosage	Time	Mon	Tues	Wed	Thurs	Fri	Sat	Sun
		A.M							
		Noon							
		P.M							
		Bedtime							

Medication	Dosage	Time	Mon	Tues	Wed	Thurs	Fri	Sat	Sun
		A.M							
		Noon							
		P.M							
		Bedtime							

Medication	Dosage	Time	Mon	Tues	Wed	Thurs	Fri	Sat	Sun
		A.M							
		Noon							
		P.M							
		Bedtime							

Medication	Dosage	Time	Mon	Tues	Wed	Thurs	Fri	Sat	Sun
		A.M							
		Noon							
		P.M							
		Bedtime							

Medication	Dosage	Time	Mon	Tues	Wed	Thurs	Fri	Sat	Sun
		A.M							
		Noon							
		P.M							
		Bedtime							

Medication	Dosage	Time	Mon	Tues	Wed	Thurs	Fri	Sat	Sun
		A.M							
		Noon							
		P.M							
		Bedtime							

Medication	Dosage	Time	Mon	Tues	Wed	Thurs	Fri	Sat	Sun
		A.M							
		Noon							
		P.M							
		Bedtime							

Medication	Dosage	Time	Mon	Tues	Wed	Thurs	Fri	Sat	Sun
		A.M							
		Noon							
		P.M							
		Bedtime							

Medication	Dosage	Time	Mon	Tues	Wed	Thurs	Fri	Sat	Sun
		A.M							
		Noon							
		P.M							
		Bedtime							

Medication	Dosage	Time	Mon	Tues	Wed	Thurs	Fri	Sat	Sun
		A.M							
		Noon							
		P.M							
		Bedtime							

Medication	Dosage	Time	Mon	Tues	Wed	Thurs	Fri	Sat	Sun
		A.M							
		Noon							
		P.M							
		Bedtime							

Medication	Dosage	Time	Mon	Tues	Wed	Thurs	Fri	Sat	Sun
		A.M							
		Noon							
		P.M							
		Bedtime							

NOTES & DAILY DETAILS

Week Start: _____

Week finish: _____

Medication	Dosage	Time	Mon	Tues	Wed	Thurs	Fri	Sat	Sun
		A.M							
		Noon							
		P.M							
		Bedtime							

Medication	Dosage	Time	Mon	Tues	Wed	Thurs	Fri	Sat	Sun
		A.M							
		Noon							
		P.M							
		Bedtime							

Medication	Dosage	Time	Mon	Tues	Wed	Thurs	Fri	Sat	Sun
		A.M							
		Noon							
		P.M							
		Bedtime							

Medication	Dosage	Time	Mon	Tues	Wed	Thurs	Fri	Sat	Sun
		A.M							
		Noon							
		P.M							
		Bedtime							

Medication	Dosage	Time	Mon	Tues	Wed	Thurs	Fri	Sat	Sun
		A.M							
		Noon							
		P.M							
		Bedtime							

Medication	Dosage	Time	Mon	Tues	Wed	Thurs	Fri	Sat	Sun
		A.M							
		Noon							
		P.M							
		Bedtime							

NOTES & DAILY DETAILS

Week Start: _____

Week finish: _____

Medication	Dosage	Time	Mon	Tues	Wed	Thurs	Fri	Sat	Sun
		A.M Noon P.M Bedtime							

Medication	Dosage	Time	Mon	Tues	Wed	Thurs	Fri	Sat	Sun
		A.M Noon P.M Bedtime							

Medication	Dosage	Time	Mon	Tues	Wed	Thurs	Fri	Sat	Sun
		A.M Noon P.M Bedtime							

Medication	Dosage	Time	Mon	Tues	Wed	Thurs	Fri	Sat	Sun
		A.M Noon P.M Bedtime							

Medication	Dosage	Time	Mon	Tues	Wed	Thurs	Fri	Sat	Sun
		A.M Noon P.M Bedtime							

Medication	Dosage	Time	Mon	Tues	Wed	Thurs	Fri	Sat	Sun
		A.M Noon P.M Bedtime							

NOTES & DAILY DETAILS

Week Start: _____

Week finish: _____

Medication	Dosage	Time	Mon	Tues	Wed	Thurs	Fri	Sat	Sun
		A.M							
		Noon							
		P.M							
		Bedtime							

Medication	Dosage	Time	Mon	Tues	Wed	Thurs	Fri	Sat	Sun
		A.M							
		Noon							
		P.M							
		Bedtime							

Medication	Dosage	Time	Mon	Tues	Wed	Thurs	Fri	Sat	Sun
		A.M							
		Noon							
		P.M							
		Bedtime							

Medication	Dosage	Time	Mon	Tues	Wed	Thurs	Fri	Sat	Sun
		A.M							
		Noon							
		P.M							
		Bedtime							

Medication	Dosage	Time	Mon	Tues	Wed	Thurs	Fri	Sat	Sun
		A.M							
		Noon							
		P.M							
		Bedtime							

Medication	Dosage	Time	Mon	Tues	Wed	Thurs	Fri	Sat	Sun
		A.M							
		Noon							
		P.M							
		Bedtime							

Week Start:
Week finish:

Medication	Dosage	Time	Mon	Tues	Wed	Thurs	Fri	Sat	Sun
		A.M							
		Noon							
		P.M							
		Bedtime							

Medication	Dosage	Time	Mon	Tues	Wed	Thurs	Fri	Sat	Sun
		A.M							
		Noon							
		P.M							
		Bedtime							

Medication	Dosage	Time	Mon	Tues	Wed	Thurs	Fri	Sat	Sun
		A.M							
		Noon							
		P.M							
		Bedtime							

Medication	Dosage	Time	Mon	Tues	Wed	Thurs	Fri	Sat	Sun
		A.M							
		Noon							
		P.M							
		Bedtime							

Medication	Dosage	Time	Mon	Tues	Wed	Thurs	Fri	Sat	Sun
		A.M							
		Noon							
		P.M							
		Bedtime							

Medication	Dosage	Time	Mon	Tues	Wed	Thurs	Fri	Sat	Sun
		A.M							
		Noon							
		P.M							
		Bedtime							

Week Start: _____

Week finish: _____

Medication	Dosage	Time	Mon	Tues	Wed	Thurs	Fri	Sat	Sun
		A.M							
		Noon							
		P.M							
		Bedtime							

Medication	Dosage	Time	Mon	Tues	Wed	Thurs	Fri	Sat	Sun
		A.M							
		Noon							
		P.M							
		Bedtime							

Medication	Dosage	Time	Mon	Tues	Wed	Thurs	Fri	Sat	Sun
		A.M							
		Noon							
		P.M							
		Bedtime							

Medication	Dosage	Time	Mon	Tues	Wed	Thurs	Fri	Sat	Sun
		A.M							
		Noon							
		P.M							
		Bedtime							

Medication	Dosage	Time	Mon	Tues	Wed	Thurs	Fri	Sat	Sun
		A.M							
		Noon							
		P.M							
		Bedtime							

Medication	Dosage	Time	Mon	Tues	Wed	Thurs	Fri	Sat	Sun
		A.M							
		Noon							
		P.M							
		Bedtime							

| Week Start: _____ |
| Week finish: _____ |

Medication	Dosage	Time	Mon	Tues	Wed	Thurs	Fri	Sat	Sun
		A.M Noon P.M Bedtime							

Medication	Dosage	Time	Mon	Tues	Wed	Thurs	Fri	Sat	Sun
		A.M Noon P.M Bedtime							

Medication	Dosage	Time	Mon	Tues	Wed	Thurs	Fri	Sat	Sun
		A.M Noon P.M Bedtime							

Medication	Dosage	Time	Mon	Tues	Wed	Thurs	Fri	Sat	Sun
		A.M Noon P.M Bedtime							

Medication	Dosage	Time	Mon	Tues	Wed	Thurs	Fri	Sat	Sun
		A.M Noon P.M Bedtime							

Medication	Dosage	Time	Mon	Tues	Wed	Thurs	Fri	Sat	Sun
		A.M Noon P.M Bedtime							

Medication	Dosage	Time	Mon	Tues	Wed	Thurs	Fri	Sat	Sun
		A.M							
		Noon							
		P.M							
		Bedtime							

Medication	Dosage	Time	Mon	Tues	Wed	Thurs	Fri	Sat	Sun
		A.M							
		Noon							
		P.M							
		Bedtime							

Medication	Dosage	Time	Mon	Tues	Wed	Thurs	Fri	Sat	Sun
		A.M							
		Noon							
		P.M							
		Bedtime							

Medication	Dosage	Time	Mon	Tues	Wed	Thurs	Fri	Sat	Sun
		A.M							
		Noon							
		P.M							
		Bedtime							

Medication	Dosage	Time	Mon	Tues	Wed	Thurs	Fri	Sat	Sun
		A.M							
		Noon							
		P.M							
		Bedtime							

Medication	Dosage	Time	Mon	Tues	Wed	Thurs	Fri	Sat	Sun
		A.M							
		Noon							
		P.M							
		Bedtime							

NOTES & DAILY DETAILS

Medication	Dosage	Time	Mon	Tues	Wed	Thurs	Fri	Sat	Sun
		A.M Noon P.M Bedtime							

Medication	Dosage	Time	Mon	Tues	Wed	Thurs	Fri	Sat	Sun
		A.M Noon P.M Bedtime							

Medication	Dosage	Time	Mon	Tues	Wed	Thurs	Fri	Sat	Sun
		A.M Noon P.M Bedtime							

Medication	Dosage	Time	Mon	Tues	Wed	Thurs	Fri	Sat	Sun
		A.M Noon P.M Bedtime							

Medication	Dosage	Time	Mon	Tues	Wed	Thurs	Fri	Sat	Sun
		A.M Noon P.M Bedtime							

Medication	Dosage	Time	Mon	Tues	Wed	Thurs	Fri	Sat	Sun
		A.M Noon P.M Bedtime							

NOTES & DAILY DETAILS

Week Start: _____

Week finish: _____

Medication	Dosage	Time	Mon	Tues	Wed	Thurs	Fri	Sat	Sun
		A.M							
		Noon							
		P.M							
		Bedtime							

Medication	Dosage	Time	Mon	Tues	Wed	Thurs	Fri	Sat	Sun
		A.M							
		Noon							
		P.M							
		Bedtime							

Medication	Dosage	Time	Mon	Tues	Wed	Thurs	Fri	Sat	Sun
		A.M							
		Noon							
		P.M							
		Bedtime							

Medication	Dosage	Time	Mon	Tues	Wed	Thurs	Fri	Sat	Sun
		A.M							
		Noon							
		P.M							
		Bedtime							

Medication	Dosage	Time	Mon	Tues	Wed	Thurs	Fri	Sat	Sun
		A.M							
		Noon							
		P.M							
		Bedtime							

Medication	Dosage	Time	Mon	Tues	Wed	Thurs	Fri	Sat	Sun
		A.M							
		Noon							
		P.M							
		Bedtime							

NOTES & DAILY DETAILS

Medication	Dosage	Time	Mon	Tues	Wed	Thurs	Fri	Sat	Sun
		A.M Noon P.M Bedtime							

Medication	Dosage	Time	Mon	Tues	Wed	Thurs	Fri	Sat	Sun
		A.M Noon P.M Bedtime							

Medication	Dosage	Time	Mon	Tues	Wed	Thurs	Fri	Sat	Sun
		A.M Noon P.M Bedtime							

Medication	Dosage	Time	Mon	Tues	Wed	Thurs	Fri	Sat	Sun
		A.M Noon P.M Bedtime							

Medication	Dosage	Time	Mon	Tues	Wed	Thurs	Fri	Sat	Sun
		A.M Noon P.M Bedtime							

Medication	Dosage	Time	Mon	Tues	Wed	Thurs	Fri	Sat	Sun
		A.M Noon P.M Bedtime							

NOTES & DAILY DETAILS

Medication	Dosage	Time	Mon	Tues	Wed	Thurs	Fri	Sat	Sun
		A.M Noon P.M Bedtime							

Medication	Dosage	Time	Mon	Tues	Wed	Thurs	Fri	Sat	Sun
		A.M Noon P.M Bedtime							

Medication	Dosage	Time	Mon	Tues	Wed	Thurs	Fri	Sat	Sun
		A.M Noon P.M Bedtime							

Medication	Dosage	Time	Mon	Tues	Wed	Thurs	Fri	Sat	Sun
		A.M Noon P.M Bedtime							

Medication	Dosage	Time	Mon	Tues	Wed	Thurs	Fri	Sat	Sun
		A.M Noon P.M Bedtime							

Medication	Dosage	Time	Mon	Tues	Wed	Thurs	Fri	Sat	Sun
		A.M Noon P.M Bedtime							

Week Start: _____

Week finish: _____

Medication	Dosage	Time	Mon	Tues	Wed	Thurs	Fri	Sat	Sun
		A.M							
		Noon							
		P.M							
		Bedtime							

Medication	Dosage	Time	Mon	Tues	Wed	Thurs	Fri	Sat	Sun
		A.M							
		Noon							
		P.M							
		Bedtime							

Medication	Dosage	Time	Mon	Tues	Wed	Thurs	Fri	Sat	Sun
		A.M							
		Noon							
		P.M							
		Bedtime							

Medication	Dosage	Time	Mon	Tues	Wed	Thurs	Fri	Sat	Sun
		A.M							
		Noon							
		P.M							
		Bedtime							

Medication	Dosage	Time	Mon	Tues	Wed	Thurs	Fri	Sat	Sun
		A.M							
		Noon							
		P.M							
		Bedtime							

Medication	Dosage	Time	Mon	Tues	Wed	Thurs	Fri	Sat	Sun
		A.M							
		Noon							
		P.M							
		Bedtime